Uropathy Unplugged

A Crowngate Publication

Uropathy Unplugged

Urine Therapy How It Works!

(A Complete Healing Kit)

For The Skeptics

The culture of taking apart what we least revere has endured through the ages. We may in certainty attempt to jettison what informs our aversion, albeit not arbitrarily. The seeming unattractiveness, regardless of the testimonies of the many that have swung in to action and are reaping the benefits, of boosting the body's immunity level with what ironically is the water of life that leads from the fear of the unknown requires encouragement, not our condemnation.

ISBN 978-978-924-556-7
234-8033942317
234-8059803390

Set and printed on acid-free paper

Disclaimer

Substantial efforts have been made to ensure that the information presented in this book is accurate. However, the reader should understand that the information provided does not constitute legal, medical or professional advice of any kind.

No Liability: This work written to enlighten is distributed in the main not essentially to discourage adherence to conventional Medicare. Any liability clauses amplified or implied in the course of dissemination are thus hereby roundly disclaimed.

Use of the product and therapy constitutes acceptance of the "No Liability" policy. If you do not agree with this policy, you are strictly precluded from the use of the therapy.

Most importantly, the author shall in no way be liable for any untoward event whatsoever (including, without limitation, consequential loss or damage) directly or indirectly arising from the application of the therapy.

Contents

1

Of The Living Spring

Do you know it is painless to dissolve through the bloodstream that goiter naturally without drugs or surgery? Do you know that with the ingestion of the auto urine, cases of diabetes have been judiciously managed and even completely cured? Do you know it is easy to break up that suspicious-looking tumour and eschew the cutting up of precious human parts with the knife known by whatever name to orthodox medicine?

Do you know that with the ingestion of the autogenously generated urine, prevention as also cure of malaria is possible? Do you know it is easy to stay in perfect health through a daily dose or regular ingestion of the fresh urine?

This submission as a result of reliable personal and sundry experiences sourced directly or indirectly of the positive usage of the yet fairly known theme of urine therapy has been documented painstakingly through the ages with the absence of little or no ambiguities.

With a brief tour of the five continents of the world via the portal of the Internet, for instance, it is easy to encounter and appraise quite astounding testimonies concerning the power and gains of the therapy revealed, by the way, to man long before the advent of modern medicine.

Conversely if there are dissenting voices to the contrary, it must be expected, albeit larger still looms the universal claim that cuts across the different strata of modern society that many are experiencing great relief from ailments that may have frustrated otherwise mightily exalted miscellaneous healthcare applications.

With the line drawn as it were between the beneficiaries and promoters of this genre of alternative medicine and the extremist postulations of, in particular, certain elements affiliated to orthodox medicine, the debate to be or not to be takes the uppermost case.

If at given instances of life's vicissitudes, many finding themselves caught at the crossroads have appointed to bask in the aura of a *sit-down-and-look* mind-set, perching on the fence as it were, it is not the best approach, all things being equal. A relevant perspective is oft-repeated that the silence of conscience when essential certainly is giving an approving nod to the passage of evil.

As a beneficiary himself of the gains accruing from deference to the lessons entrenched in the therapy, it is important to let it be known specifically on which side of the divide the author belongs. It would not auger a farthing to deny that with little or no healthcare provision in place for the generality of impoverished Africans in an economy dominated by the avarice of a selfish measly few at the top, the preponderating position is of every man for himself, God for us all.

If as is generally subscribed to that no matter the level of commitment government alone cannot meet the demands of its people at any point in time, it is yet the African peculiarity that what with inherent greed and the attendant thieving at the highest level imaginable, salvaging the poverty and by extension the health level has been made the more intractable.

Today, we may have found ourselves where we are due to the continuing mismanagement of the resources, human and natural, that God infinitely has blessed the continent with. Nevertheless, it is no use lamenting that we have spilled the milk; something just has to be done. The present goal therefore is the need to touch lives, knowing full well it is more important to have tried and recorded partial or no success than not to have tried at all.

Much that necessity is said to be the mother of all inventions, it becomes imperative therefore that we get more creative even health wise. What stops us from making the best of what we have of nature and things natural when everything else has the potentials to fail us?

This brings out the relative use to which the preventive and even curative facets of the present therapy could be put. It is indisputable that harnessed, thus ensuring judiciously in conjunction with the ever feasible sponsorship of well-meaning bodies as the WHO, all hands could come on deck to salvage the deteriorating state of the African healthcare delivery system.

To gainsay the positive aspects of not only our own trado-medicinal inheritances but also of time-tested alternatives may resemble cutting the nose to spite the face. It is a space that may be hard to fill should the positive contributions of alternative medicine be completely ignored.

The author, committed not to a partial but total realization of the need to sensitize the people to the tencts of living well through simply availing of the potentialities that abound in conformity with learning to do a few things right even if this means making do with a swig of the autogenously produced water, the urine, on a periodic basis, knows as a result of personal experience that these things do work.

In a nutshell, it is important to state in clear terms that whatever may be the nature of the despair that stares us in the face or the grinding poverty that threatens to stop the way to viable quality healthcare basic needs, nature has not denied us succor in its entity. Aptly some may have summed up that were it so divinely programmed that the air we breathe was designed as a saleable commodity, the rich would have been in a position to monopolize even this all-important element without which no man born of woman could survive. Thankfully, God is not man to discriminate who the beneficiaries of a nation's annual rainfall would be.

The onus nevertheless is on us to resolve now with an open mind to latch on to the coach en route a drive towards reenergizing of the famous African healthcare standards, acknowledging that the time definitely is requiring of more of the innovativeness of proactive elements, not the enervating overviews of cynics that are only too ready to jump in to hasty conclusions.

2

Facts and Fallacies

As a result of rebuttable prejudices attributable to long-standing ritual, the fresh urine has been taken by the generality of the human race as ordinarily body waste to be dispensed of as at when the need arises. Some who know or accustomed to the practice are expected to serve as leading lights to the many that are still in the dark have at one time or the other ended up with positional statements meant to compound even more the suffering of the disinherited masses.

It is instructive that Sir Morarji Desai, former Prime Minister of India, wrote a book on the gains of the urine therapy and did commend the use to the generality of his fellow countrymen. In an interview he gave to Dan Rather he was quoted exalting the therapy as the 'perfect medical solution for the millions of Indians who cannot afford medical treatment.' His stance could not have been associated with that of one that did not know what he was talking about. He had been an all-out practitioner of the therapy himself.

Yet several decades following the man's death a news item online, *Cameroon threatens to jail urine drinkers,* by Jane Flanagan of the Daily *Telegraph*, credited to one of Sub-Sahara Africa's

Ministers that might well have reflected his government's position on such issue of paramount importance bordering on the survival and wellbeing of the people may come in handy as a pointer to the basics of the time we live in. It could only have jolted the discerning to the reality of the African situation that there could be such a fuss about the right of an individual to what he does with himself vis-à-vis his own urine.

"Given the risks of toxicity associated with ingesting urine", Messer Urbain Olanguena Awono was quoted, "the health ministry advises against the consumption of urine and invites those who promote the practice to cease doing so or risk prosecution."

In fairness, it is not far from the truth that the safety of uropathy or urinotherapy is yet to have scientific backing. This much has been attested to by quite a number of reputable bodies such as the American Cancer Society, albeit neither has science been known to dismiss outright the efficacy of the application. Yet to the Cameroonian minister the peril of 'toxicity' appears incontrovertible.

Not content with merely stopping it at the advisory role, he had proceeded with a proviso woven round the actual prosecution of whoever is napped commending the oral use of urine to another fellow man, which falls short of barely demonstrating a tendency to repression brewing somewhere too close for comfort.

Not long ago, there was ample publicity given by the press to a statement credited to another minister of that same country making Nigeria's Prophet TB Joshua's place a 'no-go' area to Cameroonians wandering in search of spiritual and medical succor outside the country's borders. That, ostensibly, some of these needy fellow Africans might have fallen in to strange hands on any of these circuitous trips to and from the Nigerian city of Lagos, as could be the case in the best of civilized society, how judiciously the minister had concluded to make the prophet answerable and labeling him the anti-Christ?

If in trooping out to the Synagogue, Church of All

Nations, in Lagos, as do many foreign nationals without prior invitation from the prophet whose healing capability is not in doubt, what manner of diplomatese does it teach to lay the blame of a mishap befalling any of these foreigners at the foot of the man at the synagogue? Countries such as the United States, the United Kingdom and a few other EU member nations may have had cause to issue warnings to their citizens to be wary of travels to terrorist-prone regions at one time or the other. But certainly, a scathing press release in this instance to disparage the person of a respectable citizen of a friendly African country by another highly placed citizen of a neighbouring country is not only unwarranted but showcases the level of finesse and tolerance at our disposal.

Of the therapy in question, the poser is, what makes the urine use more dangerous to human health than, for instance, some of the known therapies whose continued use severally has been called to question but are still largely being permitted across the civilized world?

Surely in circulation are extra potent drugs with the primary purpose of effecting a cure or the management of isolated disease conditions of the body. It is beside the matter that in the process of application some of these drugs or therapies end up weakening and destroying other organs vital to the health and normal running of the general body system.

Take for instance the case of the crab, acknowledged as the king of all maladies and for which modern medicine is yet to find a cure, there are grave concerns within and without the medical circles as regards some of the quite debilitating therapies aimed at stemming the continued growth of abnormal cancerous cells but which impairing the health of not only the adjoining body organs, have become straight poison to the subject undergoing treatment.

There is little doubt mankind is at the precipice, marooned to say the least in a world of legalities. Unfortunately, it is not law that heals. Against such hard lines of them that are ensconced on the high pedestal, persisting revelations that are well-documented have shown that the autogenous fluid is a living spring of vivacity in no way any man-made tonic could be. Put in a nutshell, the freely ingested autogenous urine can be a builder of new tissues and, as a matter of fact, of body parts ravaged by disease.

To the author, Proverbs5:15 would always stand out as one interesting reading for all times. In one short sentence, the ancient man received unambiguously divine instruction about drinking of water running from his cistern. Of the core element, the odds of multiple interpretations need not pose a paradox. It is only true that it takes more than the physical man to have access to unimpeded appraisal of the full import of Biblical sayings and by extension all things spiritual.

Today, with growing curiosity in spite of the hard knocks of them that chose to highlight the insalubrious aspect of submission to this Biblical injunction, there are reliable findings from extensive research work carried out to ascertain the wisdom of doing so even in the face of disappointing results from orthodox medicine despite many quite commendable groundbreaking strides made by modern science.

It is not in contention that the fresh healthy urine is a creation of the food we eat. It is a revelation that the healthy urine is found to consist aside of a preponderance of urea and urea nitrogen vital energy oils, anti-oxidants, vitamins and essential elements such as *Iodine, Calcium, Potassium, Magnesium, Iron, Amino Acids, Inositol, Creatinine, Tyrosine, Lysine, Zinc, Riboflavin, Vitamin B6, Vitamin B12, Proteins, Bicarbonate, Pantothenic acid, Manganese, Melatonin,* and many more that the chemist and biochemist recommend as crucial to the well-being of the body.

Certainly, the fad has caught on in the face of little encouraging posture of some whose opinions count. The unsubstantiated conclusions about the dangerous after-effects may have received wide publicity, but strong is the belief that most proceed from the realm of imagination. A practitioner knows this is not so, and being so established is prepared to vouchsafe the priceless curative values of his therapy.

With the reluctance of the modern man to return to nature, the heat turned on the free ingestion of the urine may only have continued unabated notwithstanding the little positive results from such opposition. Human nature being what it is, it is not unusual that out of petty jealousy from too much learning, bearing in mind that not infrequently the alternative medicine man is the run-of-the-mill type, the modern physician has always looked down on the alternative medicine practitioner regardless of his successes in areas where the former has experienced a degree of helplessness. The more this falls within the range of ailments that modern medicine terms incurable the higher may be the motive to deny credit wherever due.

From this premise it is necessary to do a little digression by casting back the mind to a period in the immediate past of the race. The Yoruba that occupy a territory bordering the west coast of the Atlantic spreading through the Rainforest and farther inland to the less wooded Savannah are renowned for a strong tradition of herbal medicine that rarely leaves anything to chance. A highly innovative race, the place of the herbal remedy as grounded mainly in indigenous Medicare for most ailments and disease conditions long before the contact with white influence needs no stressing.

Up till the succeeding years of the last World War, it was the practice to hang in the traditional Yoruba home aside of other strange-looking paraphernalia associated with good health and the need for self-preservation a bottle that overtime had gathered soot above the fireplace. It is cow urine for consumptive children. It was supposed to be so potent a concoction that it was sparingly administered to the sick child. Eventually, the fad being frowned upon by modern medicine saw it completely taken off the list of traditional medication. There is, nonetheless, little doubt it had served its purpose at the time.

Certainly, the horror could well have been imagined if by any strange twist of mind an internal application of one's urine that was far more superior to the cow urine had actually been openly prescribed as an antidote for certain ailments at the time. This is not a blanket statement that the practice was absolutely unheard of but that the very few that might have resorted out of desperation to the use for sure could be said to have been on their own.

Against such a background it was more than a pleasant surprise for the author to learn as a young man leafing one morning through the publication, *The Sunday Tribune,* that autogenous urine freely taken could not only make for quite robust health, but also could be a complete cure for a series of diseases, no matter the name or characteristics. Coming from a paper, a brainchild of the sage Awo and published by the African Newspapers of Nigeria, which has been described by CAC Pastor Gabriel Makinwa as the 'light of the world', the mark of authenticity was not in doubt.

The article based on a book authored by the then India's Prime Minister, Morarji Desai, was quite an eye-opener and had set the young man on a frantic search for a copy that had seemed then like looking for water in the desert. I was later to discover that some Indian tribes and Eskimos had as a matter of fact cultivated the habit of drinking their own urine and in a long while remained healthy for doing so.

I may as well add hereby how an elderly friend of mine to whom I thought to divulge this secret of inexpensively maintaining a perfect health had actually taken me by surprise by revealing to me how his mother when bathing them had had the knack of inducing him and his brother to pee in the cup of her hand, and which fresh urine she usually gave them to drink.

It is worth knowing that much as the writer is not an advocate of self-medication and neither is he out to discredit any of the popular patented drugs on the shelves the world over, the free-flowing fluid is not only credited with being invaluable in combating minor ailments with absolutely no side effects, but also the so-called terror king and before which orthodox medicine has been hopelessly outwitted.

Now, what with the endless assertions of answers to different diseases plaguing humanity that daily flood the marketplace, the need to be circumspect in embarking on any form of therapy no matter the rosy promises cannot be discountenanced. It can only be expected that great caution is made the key word where one's life and the overall wellbeing of the body are involved.

Many thanks to several pioneers for extensive research works and salutary labours at the service of humanity, even in such extreme cases where surgical intervention may appear the only way out for modern medicine, the therapy could and actually is reputed to have performed astonishingly to save precious lives and nip in the bud needless suffering of the human body.

3

The Therapeutic Values

Following a popular survey carried out by the Chinese News agency, it came to light that several millions of Chinese wake up every morning to take their urine.

Not only were these Chinese accustomed to washing and thereby protecting the skin of their young babies with urine, the curative values of making do with especially the stuff pissed by underage boys for long had proved irresistible. That the practice is still largely in vogue till the present day only an unguided tour of the countryside may readily reveal.

In India it is a long-established fact that a large percentage of Indians take their urine and so do the Eskimos. Today Europeans and Americans are learning to drink of their urine and so soon it has become a fad that people are turning daily to their urine.

Why do you think they do this? Certainly, they are not short of creative thinking, or are they? One answer may suffice, and that is, the world has always learned the tricks of allowing nature to intervene when necessary, especially where the human health is concerned, notwithstanding the giant strides made by science.

Now, the urine unaffectedly has been described as

waste that is voided as at when due because the body has no need of it. This is not only from the layman's point of view but some that are supposed to know but for reason of mischief pretends even this to be so. However, as stated in the earlier portion of work, urine that invariably consists of whatever nourishment the body takes needs be seen in a much clearer light than this. .

There is little to add but that the stuff in question is too precious to be wasted the way we do, ignorant of the cost in so doing. Not only is it a simple means to sound health, the use of the urine has been found to be a dependable therapy in the cure of some rather deadly diseases no matter the name or characteristics.

The fresh urine has a wide range of vitamins and salt nutrients that are of great benefit to the body, aside of the urea that though toxic is found to be of no side effect in the process of oral re-absorption into the system.

If the injunction in Proverb 5:15 advocating the free ingestion of one's cistern predated modern science with its loads of findings and laudable achievements including oftentimes the junks, then the earlier conclusion that urine is body waste that should be discountenanced could only have stemmed from a pool of long-held prejudices. Without doubt, the ingestion of one's urine is an assured way of maintaining robust health less the hassles. As a preventive and insurance against ill-health, it is a practice with origin traceable to old times.

If long made popular by the Indians and also the Chinese, whose population put together is a large chunk off the sum total of what constitutes obedience to the creator's bid for man to multiply and replenish the earth, then the life-preserving qualities may require more than the lip service the world of science tends to accord it. This is more so seeing it is a most effective way of tackling the scourge of diseases that otherwise has proved intractable even in the face of science and the technological advancement of time.

Indeed, the stuff in focus has long been known to serve the dual purpose of keeping the body healthy whilst ensuring that the pangs of hunger are kept at bay for as long as possible. Marooned at sea, sailors that survived the harrowing experience of shipwrecks had done so solely on their urine even as they watched their comrades that scoffed at the practice give up the ghost.

As a form of nature-cure, the simplicity of administration must have endeared it principally to many in the past as indeed to the modern man not excluding the city-dweller enshrined in his complexities.

If to the Christians the application has Biblical authority, it is no less significant that the Hindus accorded it a quite larger-than-life status of propitious water of the Hindu god Lord Shiva. As a matter of fact, the ingestion of the stuff was a pre-condition to serious meditational heights by adherents of the Hindu religion.

In Islam the place of the wisdom of so fortifying the body, call it immunity enhancement, is neither void. The words of the prophet reechoed in a portion of the six Hadith collections, the Sahih Bukhari, in Sunni Islam. Mohammed was severally quoted handing out specific instructions to his followers of the time to avail of the medicinal benefits of drinking of the camel urine, which is even of less quality to the human stuff, all for one purpose, the health of the human body, knowing full well a man has but one body at a time in one lifespan.

The effectiveness of the therapy promoted by the few to the present age thus has never been in doubt despite the reservations of them that perceive it as intrinsically mere filth.

Way back in the 17th century French women of the aristocratic class were reputed to delight in enhancing the beauty of their skin by bathing with their urine. Sir Morarji Desai, Prime Minister of India, who as a believer and practitioner of the kind of therapy and known to have commended its use to the generality of his countrymen and through his work on the same subject to the world at length, had passed on at 99.

As the nature-cure exemplar and author, the worthy JW Armstrong indicated unequivocally in his book, *The water of Life,* impeded urination and venereal diseases, growths and tumors said to be cancerous, as also cataracts, kidney and chronic skin infections have been known to yield way quickly.

It is the more remarkable in that the system involved is so simple that the ordinary man in the street or the housewife in the most backward areas of civilization can undertake the therapy with success as could the city dweller and they of the elitist class. That the urine ingested orally and sometimes through external applications could actually course through those arteries and veins to isolate and perform the healing of diseased areas of the body even where mutilation may have been recommended could not but beat the imagination.

It is only natural that being powerless in the face of what could have been but a deliberate design of the master builder Himself, some have attempted to ascribe the phenomenon to faith healing. But, as the worthy John Armstrong has rightly affirmed, it is more than mere faith healing. Not only do the lower animal species benefit as much as humans do, but considerable results were recorded when applied in the case of layer birds.

Yet if remarkable successes have been recorded in various cases of infections, pneumonia, hepatitis, renal failure, psoriasis and so on, it does not imply that the application in every known disease condition could be said to have met with the same degree of success in every case. Many diabetic and severe arthritic conditions, for instance, may have proved to be among the quite stubborn exceptions. A case of the arthritic condition of an old colleague and friend readily comes to mind. He used to be a strong fellow and rather quite conscious of the mass of hard muscles on every limb as a service man. By the time we were reunited after about a decade of separation he was almost a physical wreck. A sight to behold, every application of orthodox medicine having failed to effect a cure and with constant pains racking his body, to him simple locomotion had become such a burden. Unfortunately, uropathy when the author introduced it to him was also of no use. Notwithstanding, the naturalness involved of the whole process is enough to have stirred the spirit of the adventurous.

Interestingly, positive results from the application in some otherwise quite unusual disease conditions oftentimes have been rather stunning. Many cases that have been otherwise given up for lost have been turned round in a simple manner that could not but leave even the discerning bowled over.

Soon after the success with a diabetic condition, this author surfaced in one of the military cantonments in Lagos midway through the year (2009) and had the opportunity of giving a sick soldier a free consultancy service concerning some rather suspicious looking growth in the neck. The sergeant, who was diabetic, had been bed-ridden at the Military Hospital for some time and was expected to return to the hospital for an operation to excise the growth. Sitting in the left side of the neck, it was almost as big as a fist and, if anything, had been one source of constant anxiety to the man and his family.

I suggested a urine fast, urine pack and massage

of patient's body excluding the affected area. In a short period the abnormal growth disappeared completely leaving no trace behind. The success was astounding; the enlargement had dissolved completely through the bloodstream and up till date without any side-effect.

Another soldier known to the author was soon placed on the same kind of treatment by the first patient and at the time of compiling the first edition of the earlier work on diabetes, his own condition had improved considerably. It is strange nevertheless that both serving soldiers had been through various degrees of diabetic conditions. Has diabetes, how remotely, anything in common with any form of growth or abnormal enlargement of the body, malign or benign?

Maybe we need not indulge ourselves nor raise the hopes of sufferers of all manner of diseases that the therapy could be the cure-all for every disease condition. The case of a certain lady close to the author may serve as a good example. She had remained barren for as long as two decades or thereabouts. Following the success with another woman who preferred the therapy than a visit to the herbalist, I thought I could be of help and inquired what the matter was. According to her doctor, she was diagnosed with 'ovulatory infertility'. I suggested to her the therapy. I have no way of knowing if she ever followed the steps recommended faithfully, all I knew is that she had remained barren even till today.

A fellow from the air force once asked at a seminar venue if actually there could not be hope for HIV/AIDS carriers with the range of testimonies that abound attesting to the reality of uropthay as agent of healing. One question that did not take the resource person unawares, seeing as the possibility of finding a cure along that line had occurred ever often and to him in all his waking moments, however, it is only necessary to try and relay clearly what I told the guy and this is to the effect that such an experimentation if feasible is certainly not what the present scope is all about. It is not unlikely that something spectacular may crop up later that could astound the world in the near future. Presently, with the endless list of spurious claims to cure for as many disease conditions as are under the sky including HIV/AIDS by specifically every quack that would want to be seen as a healer of sorts, mum definitely would be the word.

4

Nature's Healing Agent

AS in every other thing, several application theories have been advanced, some of which may appear ludicrous. While it is not essential to refute or fail to acknowledge whatever distinction may have constituted the background to the regime prescribed in each individual practice or orientation, it is the author's opinion that simple would do. A rather complex approach in order to be seen as enhancing the simple instruction concerning the ingestion of the stuff produced autogenously may not be necessary.

There are supposed to be no airs of mysticism or any recourse to high-sounding technicalities in packaging the knowledge involved to arrive at needed results. The entire process is as simple as ABC. Where some manner of alternative therapies comes with quite complex methodology and others with gadgets and things, uropathy as propounded overtime is devoid of all this.

Such stuffs as diluting the urine and starting with a few drops at a time to a measure of warm or sterile water are ordinarily uncalled for. Whilst simple and straightforward application would suffice, some local source had tried to advocate allowing the urine to settle and after which the patient should add edible salt and things to a fluid that came ordinarily fortified with an ample supply of salt nutrients in their natural form.

It is interesting to note that the advocate of a regime of rigorous massage aside of the oral use of the fresh urine, hinges the logic on the express need of the patient for additional form of nourishment especially where a long fasting period is being observed. The body rubs ensure friction that opens up the pores of the skin naturally, he propounds. It is thus to the body's benefits that the urine through the skin may find further inroad to fortify the body undergoing the chastising of short or long fast.

For preventive purposes and maintenance of top

immunity level it is enough to note that waking up early in the morning and quaffing all that is voided in terms of quantity and quality serves the most use. The constancy of application depends more on each individual's preference. This author, who as a child hated herbal concoctions, even in adulthood had had the least inclination to medicinal compulsion. Yet romancing the stuff on an on-and-off basis, as he was to find out, had in no way affected the overall health condition of the body, and in particular with reference to the BP and blood sugar that continued to remain normal.

What is quite important and this as much as the therapy itself is ensuring that one maintains a close tab on what one eats even when the inclination to touch the therapy is not there. It is, however, not the best approach to abstain from one's daily dosage especially the early morning shot for longer than necessary.

Whatever is the reason why one would want to embark on taking one's urine that by convention is adjudged taboo, I have always enjoined the would-be practitioner to start with a well-managed short fast followed by a fairly longer fasting period in the case of a stubborn disease condition.

By a well-managed fast what this author implies centres on the modus operandi. The correct process is essential in the management of a fast at all times even when it has little to do with the type of cleansing recommended for this purpose.

Significantly, the beginning and close of the fast must be rightly observed. Both aspects are important if one is to derive immediate and maximum benefits there from. It is not as if it's the fasting with or without the fresh urine that matters, but the technique has been found to be quite effective and thus highly recommended by the author.

That there is no magic in a piece of meat taken between the teeth only to disappear down the gullet everyone must by now be aware. In the absence of the least form of complications or long-winded explaining to do, it requires no shaving of specialty or pretences, to achieving the desired effect. The mere ingestion of the fluid had worked in time past and would continue to work whatever is anyone's position to the contrary.

It is not about faith-healing, one may be a raving non-conformist or an atheist that scoffs at the existence of God, and it would still work fine. If, however, from the incurable cynicism of man some have postulated to narrow down its effectiveness to faith-healing, it is but common sense that horses, goats cats and no less dogs have reportedly equally received maximum benefits as much as man.

The beauty of it is that no known side effects have been documented even if applied in a kid or the septuagenarian and whoever. The miracle, if we may so imply, is how the common urine that is freely dispensed by man all over the place, could following ingestion easily course through the internal organs and hidden conduit pipes to carry out the healing and even renewal of tissues and body parts wasted through the passage of illness. In this alone man needs to ponder and in an aside learn to give glory to the heavens that these things have been found to be so.

So, a lot of claims, some falling barely short of divine intervention, have been made to authenticate the efficacy of the therapy. While this author is not out to disprove these claims nor lay undue emphasis on the power of the therapy, it is nevertheless safe to restrict the veracity of the healing power and success to direct experiences within one's sphere of influence in the meantime. It may not be a surprise that experts in various fields related to no less orthodox medicine have at one time or the other made known their findings with respect to oftentimes astonishing successes where modern medicine have met the brick wall. This may be the exception; the larger majority would prefer to keep mum where attempts to disparage the practice have yielded little results.

Meanwhile, the fact that with his earlier work on the application of the therapy, the author has chosen to demonstrate in plain language that it is possible with a combination of fasting and the urine to dissolve quite naturally the goiter, while also reversing a diabetic condition, does not mean that the method enthused is the rule.

The experimentation with the maladies in the said work, *How I Defeated Diabetes Without Drugs,* and from which copious passages have been lifted, may appear to suffice based on what had been a stereotype. Nonetheless, it is a tested and outstanding approach and one to which the author freely subscribes. The fact remains, however, that in general, as is universally acknowledged, numerous are the paths that lead to the marketplace.

A fellow the author ran across at the office of a busy city press early in the year 2010 readily volunteered the airing of his own wonderful experience with regards to the therapy. He had been hospitalized with complications from diabetes and with blood sugar level shooting up close to 300 mg/dl, he was fed with amongst other things a high dosage of glucophate and at the end of the day returned home still quite sick, having shed but very little of the blood sugar.

At home someone had hinted of the realness of the therapy for him to combine the drinking of his water with a diet rich in bran, beans, spinach, oily fish, and plantain flour. He never added the fast but cut his intake of alcohol and aerated water. He eschewed red meat and ate sparingly of chicken stripped of the skin. At the end of a couple of weeks his sugar level dropped to 85 mg/dl. A young man, he had since redoubled as a worker in the vineyard of the Lord and at the time we met in robust health.

About a decade prior to the publication of the book on diabetes, the author discovered by chance that the so-called crisis made popular in cases of sickle-cell anemia condition could actually extend to the menstrual circle. Why, towards the end of the last millennium there was this woman friend in the throes of a menstrual crisis, an occurrence that customarily preceded the beginning of the flow since the very first day she experienced the event as a young girl. In her late twenties and yet to be a mother, the expression of quiet horror on her face was such to suggest she must have had a spiritual bout with the devil himself.

I'd breezed in to the flat and there she was in the sitting-room, her hair disheveled and a forlorn look on her face where she sat spread-eagled on the carpet. Maybe I am putting it mildly but, honestly, to pretend I'd seen something like that before may amount to an untruth. Incidentally, this is a young woman who had always believed in me. She had often repeated herself that I seemed to know about virtually everything. Yet it is no use to claim to know what one does not know.

Somehow I must have succeeded in calming her

down and later told her about the therapy and fast, the option that could not fail. I could still recall the look of shock and repulsion in her face the day leading by example I'd quaffed all that I voided one morning to show her how harmless drinking one's urine was. Thank God, she also gave it a try and as we fasted together it was the last time that she experienced the ever recurring trauma of a fitful menstrual circle.

At about the same period, I found myself in company of two young women in a restaurant one afternoon when the topic of childlessness came up. One of the ladies was an old friend and the other who joined us later at the dining table was newly married. Before I knew it, there followed a spirited discussion in which different theories were advanced as to the cause of infertility and even impotence in the men folks. When the younger woman who had been married to her heartthrob for barely a year confided in her friend concerning her inability to retain the man's sperm at intercourse despite several medications and visits to the doctor and her friend promised to take her to some herbalist, I dropped the hint of some time-tested alternative that had never failed and subsequently introduced the therapy.

It must have been all that she had been waiting for. She'd never had cause to visit the herbalist in all her life, she said, and thus quickly latched on to the urine option. At the end of a short weekend fast, the seemingly stubborn condition became history and she took in thereafter without hassles.

Following the success with the diabetes, I ran in to a certain lady during the early morning jogging hour. She seemed to have left it too late before embarking on that not-too useful hard program to shed the excess load of fat and flesh; she was overweight in every respect.

A top company executive in her prime, it was pitiable to hear her open up soon after we became jogging partners and I had observed aloud how extremely fat she had looked. So I'd suggested a fast on her urine, thus following what must have been the initial distaste, which was only to be expected, before long she was on the way to shedding the excess weight while she looked extremely delectable.

Her case that was not much different from the story of this other lady who though barely in to her thirties looked so matronly to have created the impression of one in the middle age, has proved beyond any reasonable doubt that it is easy with a little self-discipline and a fast on one's urine to keep in perfect shape even where the body over the years has accumulated a great deal of fat.

It is easy to go on and on. 2005 saw me relocate briefly to Ibadan, the heartland of Nigeria's southwest. There was a certain lady that worked in one of the banks in Allen at the city centre. Of course, there is no way one could have ignored her presence, more so as she lived directly in the adjoining house that was a nightly rendezvous for a group of lively beer-quaffing men, including the friend and I. A pretty and convivial creature, nonetheless she had a ring of telltale blisters around her handsome neck.

Now, the day she came home earlier than usual and related the story of how 'the soldiers' held up transactions in her bank throughout the day, we came round to getting a little interested in each other. Alarmed that even Nigerian soldiers, famous for their great docility, could now decide to take the laws in to their hands because salaries were not paid on time, I tried to extract from her the details, only to discover the soldiers she was talking about were actually the retirees whose pensions had been late in coming.

For her pains, I asked to know what she was doing about the eruption that had formed a ring round her neck, a condition which I suspected must have been the outcome of the constant friction from her imitation gold necklace against the bleaching stuff she, as indeed most ladies, delighted on. Her medications having failed her, I suggested she saved some of her urine in a small container for a few days after which she could commence to apply it to the spot day and night before her bath. In the shortest time imaginable the blisters disappeared completely, leaving the skin on the neck of our lady friend almost as silky as the skin of a small baby.

Not long after my return to the country in the new year, I'd resurfaced at the Ikeja Army Cantonment and was astonished that another soldier who'd had a long bout with tuberculosis had quite recently lighted on the therapy. He had stuck strictly to taking his urine, everything he voided daily, to the exclusion of a formal fast, having, as a matter of fact, received no direct instruction to include the fast but got cured completely of the disease.

We may well afford to bring this chapter to a close but maybe after a little further admonition concerning the necessity of early detection of disease conditions to ensure early attention to whatever may be the ailment plaguing the system. This is the more necessary in order to avoid needless complications not only with respect to the therapy under focus but invariably where every healthcare application is concerned.

It is not uncommon that the culture of periodic checkup of the body system from visits to the hospitals is lacking in the developing world. The few that adhere to this regimen are the privileged, the rich or service personnel and those in government or corporate employ that are by tradition compelled to undergo annual system checkups. Yet the gains of such periodic visits even when there is the least suspicion of impending danger to the body system are enormous. It aids early detection of impaired body organs, making it easier for the body in need of attention to attune effortlessly to external corrective measures and heal itself. More so, it enhances not just the preventive aspect, which being the central theme of in particular this treatise, is paramount, but also the curative promises thereof.

Now, if the urge to go out there on the street corner sometimes to let people know the power in the fresh urine before long was threatening to border on what might resemble a passion, to the author it was more of a given opportunity to touch lives. There is the quote that runs to the effect that

‘When you have something great you share it with the world.’

It is thus with soul pride he takes it up to announce how it made his day when at the tail-end of putting together the first edition of the first book he received the news one quiet evening that the other service man with the growth in the neck was actually already at Katsina in the northern part of the country on his way to the UN mission area at Darfur. A gallant soldier as they come, his voice rang true with excitement as he relayed across the line in response to the author’s inquiry concerning his health, ‘Alhamudududullahi! My health has been perfectly restored, and ‘am on my way to Darfur, sir!'

Nothing could have been quite heart-warming than knowing this thing actually works. If then reliable statistics have it that nationals of diverse nations across the globe wake up in the morning and taste of their own water and have remained in robust health for so doing in a long while, one can only hope the present effort to promote the culture this side of creation yields requisite dividends in record time.

5

Miscellanies

There is no gainsaying the truth that the best liquid for the effective functioning of the body and body organs would always be water. It is essential that after waking up from sleep each morning one takes a glass of or two of cool, clean water. If, however, for whatever reasons, any liquid other than this is desirable, then the autogenous fluid as soon as it is passed can only serve as the better option.

It aids the bowel movement and in turn enhances blood circulation. With the cleansing of the belly and internal organs, it acts as tonic preparing the body for the day's activities.

It is extremely unhealthy that due to constipation, for instance, the body's elimination process is in anyway hampered. Nothing therefore could have sounded as odd as the story given publicity recently in one of the dailies that for some rather peculiar reasons a man whose picture was emblazoned on the front page attended to his toilet demands once in a week! This author recognizes that what with a regular dose of his water first thing immediately after bed every morning the situation could have been easily reversed if not absolutely impossible.

Concerning the ingestion of one's water, there is no better way than the simple one of taking it the very minute it is voided. It works!

For the purpose of maintaining a perfect health without recourse to (too many) synthetic substances including matters that invariably are useless to the body or, simply, to eschew needless spending on drugs and keep at bay parasitic professionals for as far as possible, there is nothing like one's urine taken first thing in the morning and with additional swigs through the day and the eventide. The authority would have the author believe he took all that his body produced.

Yes, the early morning shot for the body is unlike anything that follows after in both quantity and quality. The system even while the body is in a state of rest has undergone overnight a process of chemical rejuvenation, a progressive replacement of much of the vigor expended in the course of living through the day. And with an additional prospect of escaped hormones vital to the wellbeing of the system trapped in the healthy urine following a normal night rest, there is hardly anything that touches the early morning stuff in richness.

Now, in passing, it is but natural that the waste be flushed out at the completion of each circle of extraction of what the body needs from the abundance of ingested nutrition day-by-day. In this, the body needs be assisted to carry out efficiently its assignment. This the urine does without side effects aside of constituting on its own strength an immune-booster, leaving the body refreshed, light, and the owner as fit as a fiddle all day.

It has been proved that the taste of the healthy urine depends more on the type of nutrition that passes through the system; any one feeling so inclined no matter where he stands can only come up with independent findings to corroborate this. It follows to say the accumulated fluid overnight as indeed what the body generates in a single day is much more than mere residue that the bladder is anxious to expel but a concentration of bits and pieces which, subjected to the probing of science, have not failed to impress the science world and whoever may have entertained opinions that are at variance with the claims of the immeasurable therapeutic values to mankind by enthusiasts.

As a preventive therefore against the occurrence or reoccurrence, as it may be, of needless and avoidable ailments, the urine is incomparable. For the purpose of healing, however, the therapy as earlier mentioned could be said to optimize its rather astounding successes in combination with a fast, short or otherwise, depending on the nature of the malady.

A methodical abstinence with regards to food or the tendency to clog the system with yet more food when actually not needed such as at the juncture of a dilemma is advocated. It is to the human understanding that the sick dog would rather shun its food and resort instead to nibbling at grasses and herbs by instinct till the threat facing it is over. Food to the critically ill at this stage that tends to be injurious may be ill-advised.

The external rubbing of old urine for as long as two hours or thereabouts is advocated. As an additional impetus to good results, it is an exercise laden with distinct potentialities. It lowers the pangs of hunger as much as helping to fight palpitation during especially protracted fasting period. The important areas to note are the face, the neck and the feet. It is a revelation that the hands that massage the body tend to be as soft as a newborn baby's, the fluid being without doubt the skin food for all times and indeed all skin types.

The place of the urine is even more than what has yet been given credit by most enthusiasts. This author discovered early in his experimentation that old urine could be made to perform as much wonders as shampoo and with no known side effects aside of the stench.

To put to rest the morbid fear of bumps after that usual visit to the hair salon, it is safe to keep old urine as handy as ever in a bathroom corner. I recommend its use as after-shave for its soothing effect; it leaves the skin smooth and fresh even when no soap is employed to bathe the face after.

The wonders of the urine in tackling ailments and improving on impaired human organs may not be as apparent save to them that are honored with a first-hand experience. To sufferers from wounds that simply refused to heal or scars and eruptions left on the skin as a result of prolonged contact with body ornaments and things, a treat with the urine over a brief period had done the miracle to victims to whom the author recommended its usage one time or another.

A former soldier who by accident of mutual work experience had warmed his way in to the heart of the author on one of the unending rounds of annual pensions paper stuff had fallen sick. He was dying by installments, as the award-wining world-acclaimed stage artiste, Duro Ladipo of *Oba Koso* fame, once put it just before he finally passed on. The author was shocked running in to Ole Sol one evening. Ole Sol, as he loved to be addressed by the rest of the community where he lived, was bent double hanging on tightly to a walking-stick. Old soja never die, is a fond saying midst the veterans. But here was the merry fellow himself looking just too good to go! Of course, they constitute the neglected members of society who in the words of a former President qualify for death as a result of old age. And talk of the bland look of the face; it is just about the right sign of a figure at the dismal point of existence. It is enough to hold government responsible that such as these are lacking in any form of state-sponsored medical provision, and what with the monthly stipend by the state disproportionately at variance with, for instance, the largesse committed to erstwhile militants that only a little while ago ganged up to rain down fire and brimstone on the fatherland.

So there was the Arty guy that saw it happen and

could still tell you how many ordinances were fired in the taking of which rebel stronghold of heroic Biafra looking decrepit almost like a retired farmer devastated by long bouts of arthritic pains.

Wandering what could have happened in barely three months that we last met, I was quick in pumping him for the details of this ailment that so soon was threatening to disarm and make POW our unsung hero. That the nature of the sickness was cloaked in the usual medical parlance earmarked to mesmerize even the patient about whom it was written there was no doubt. Yet the last thing on his mind was death, Old Sol still had it in him to want to give life another try. Of course, it is a fact that not even the oldies want to die; everyone would rather stay alive whatever the circumstance of age. So it was even with our man, the hero of many a battle who seeing there was little hope for him dependent on the State General Hospital facilities, paid an amount totaling up to twenty thousand naira to one of the country's Chinese medicine entrepreneurs who had charged him Naira Sixty Thousand for his services inclusive of computer scanning of his body system and prescriptions subsequently of herbal capsules from China homeland.

Asked if there was any marked improvement in his condition following the payment of the said amount to his doctor, his response was an emphatic no. Naturally, there was nothing to hide;

it was there all right for the eyes to see.

I could not conceal the feeling of distrust of his 'doctor' in spite of the confidence reposed by the patient in the unknown animal man with his scanning gadgets and things. It was nauseating to behold the once buoyant soldier conclude in a voice unlike him that perhaps his recovery would come no sooner than he could beat the constraint of scarce funds to offset the balance.

So we had a rather long talk and at the end of which I briefed him concerning the possibilities of trying the urine therapy. A brave fellow, he agreed to give it a try immediately. I didn't fail to inform him of the need to avoid staining his urine with alcoholic drinks and to suspend the use of other medications including what the herbal networker gave him.

Being a Muslim for whom fasting was mandatory, he took it in good faith the suggestion that he commenced with a short fast and later a not-so-short fast after which he could suffice on his normal everyday feeding habit in addition to drinking everything that he voided.

At the end of the month there was Ole Sol without the walking-stick bounding up the street. He beamed with vigour as he came. His level of all-round fitness must have surpassed his own initial expectations. I had suggested to him a regime of early morning exercise the type he was used to while in the service. The gains showed easily. With the radiance on his soon rejuvenated face, one knew without being told the combination had worked incredibly well

Now, it is noteworthy that if those on the other side of the divide that could ill-afford to face the prohibitive costs of seeking medical attention in private hospitals or make the many rounds of overseas trips to specialists hospitals are tailored by condition to weather the storm even as guinea pigs in all sorts of outlandish experimentation, not so the rich who having all the funds at their disposal elect to make periodic tours of the best hospitals abroad for minor aches and routine check-ups. It is only to be expected that the latter set would frown mightily at the mere mention of the therapy and take off in alarm, careless the regular treatment on account of which they coughed out exorbitant fees was not fail proof.

A story told online once ran to the effect that an apparently frustrated Indian doctor who in a state of complete helplessness contrived to repackage and introduce as safe drugs the urine samples submitted on request by some quite wealthy clients of his. To the relief of the chief protagonist of this real life drama, the Oga-Madame whose ailing conditions every other prescription had failed to correct received spontaneously their healing.

Now, if the doctor being clever not by half got

paid for his services and Oga-Madame received their healing, the lesson essentially is not about the autogenous urine that cured the maladies but that the wealthy would always pay fat sums even for their own urine surreptitiously dispensed as drug!

At this juncture, it is appropriate to endeavour to bring up the story of two retired RSMs of the army both very dear to me, good soldiers, by any standards well-suited for the job at every turn of the way.

One of the former RSMs was a hard drinker. It is not a secret that many used to be as young soldiers but while some managed to call it quits in time, others simply could not.

The second RSM was a devout Muslim and one of those who had called off the pact with the bottle on time. Prior to the publication of the first edition of work on diabetes management without drugs, and which was not much of a book, anyway, I ran into the latter that I initiated promptly in to the cult of disciples of uropathy. His enthusiasm that way back in uniform could be infectious now was even something else. In no time he had bought in to the intricacies of the therapy that hardly did a day pass that we did not devote enough time to exchange ideas on the phone. He is still alive and very much in good health.

I had used the occasion of the subsequent reunion of the comrades-in-arms at the barracks to give away complimentary copies of the then recently printed report, *How I defeated Diabetes Without Drugs,* to some of the men including the RSM that still cherished his drink. He threw it away, no doubt about that. Six months later the news spread that he had passed on.

Now, it makes quite interesting reading that a source along the line suggests for the female to clean up properly before collecting the water for drinking. It may not sound unreasonable to stress the subject of cleanliness much as it is like man to wonder what that aspect of hygiene got to do with it. Maybe the nature of urine makes it ordinarily an all-inclusive antiseptic. Notwithstanding, it is fundamental that utmost consideration be given to how one handles the stuff. After all, it is an old saying that cleanliness is next to Godliness.

Not strangely, the source is silent on suchlike preconditions for the men folks. Oh well, since about every birth occurs at the hospital or government certified maternity homes in modern times, the sight of one uncircumcised male child with the possibility of accumulated dirt and viral infection could not but stand out as the exception - unlike in the past when some of the boys from the other faith shocked you to the marrow displaying about the place untidy-looking foreskins like no one's business!

The author

Isola Adeabayoa Alabi is a nature-cure enthusiast, a prolific writer, and an Internet marketing consultant. He lives in Lagos, the financial capital of the West African sub-region.

Other books by the author include:
A Holistic Approach To A Healthy Lifestyle
How I Defeated Diabetes Without Drugs
The Diminishing Order of Yoruba Ritual Drama

For further reading see:

Urine therapy

From Wikipedia, the free encyclopedia

For Health News join The Author @

www.cgatelink.com.ng/

www.ingramcontent.com/pod-product-compliance
Ingram Content Group UK Ltd.
Pitfield, Milton Keynes, MK11 3LW, UK
UKHW061706190726
13853UKWH00008B/2432

9 789789 245567